How I Lost 50 Pounds in Six Months

by Dylan Murray

direct email:
dylansebooks@gmail.com

website:
www.dylanonline.com

Facebook Page:
https://www.facebook.com/50pounds6months

Facebook Group (The Best Choice!):
https://www.facebook.com/groups/1641314272806119/

For Andrea,
who got me moving this body

And Kim,
who got me writing this book

Table of Contents

An Introduction That *Might* be Worth Reading
Full Disclosure
The Timeframe
Growing Bigger and Bigger
Then 30 Happened
Aren't I Special?
Exercise
Life is not a Pie Eating Contest
Where Does the Fat Go?
Exercise is a Habit
All the Extras
Using the Scale
Food Tracking
Skinny People and Calories
Types of Calories
Food and Recipes
Meal Planning
Sleep
Getting Started (and Losing the Weight)
The Fallout
Sample Calorie Count
Basal Metabolic Rate Examples

An Introduction That *Might* be Worth Reading

So to be fair, I started writing this ebook twelve weeks into the six month plan. At that point, I hadn't lost 50 pounds yet; but I had lost about about 25 pounds in 12 weeks. I seemed to have landed on a plan that worked.

As it turns out, I was right. I started in May. (To be completely accurate, I probably started ten years ago.) But in May, I decided to go at my weight problem with the full force of science and math. (Crazy, right?) It's November, and I am down 50 pounds.

At 50 pounds lighter, I don't have a new lease on life. I don't spring out of bed ready to write a novel, record an album, and sing in a local choral group. I am still struggling. I don't love exercising. I still have problems controlling my eating habits at night. And while I look thinner, I don't have a huge boost in self confidence. I am still me, and the hard work I put into the last six months has not made me into a brand new man.

However, the mental anguish is gone. I was out to dinner with some friends, and one woman brought a date -- a Swedish man I had never met. Throughout the course of the meal we talked about food and wine. We talked about exercise. We talked about hiking up the big hill to see the little church in Marseille, France. And not once, did I think that he was looking at me with pity.

Prior to the weight loss, I would have held back on participating. I would have thought the new friend was thinking, "Oh poor Dylan. I'll be it was hard for him to walk up that hill." (Or however you would say that in Swedish.) And after the meal, when everyone stripped down to their skivvies and jumped in the water, I didn't hide in the corner and sneak into the water. I just happily participated.

So my diet and weight loss hasn't made me a new man. But it's made me, me again.

Full Disclosure

I have plenty of time for this process. I work from home in a foreign city populated by a distant and judgemental people (the French). I don't have many social activities, and I make most of my own meals.

"Why aren't you eating out in France?" you ask. Because I'd like to lose weight. And I am tired of blase waitresses antsy for a smoke break.

I have the time to prepare meals, exercise, and sleep. Each being a pillar of this scheme that seems to allow me to drop weight after ten years of wondering why I couldn't even fit into my former "heavy" clothes.

I don't have a lot of money to invest in this diet. No trainers or expensive diet shakes. I don't have a membership to a gym, and I don't own overpriced treadmills that can read my pulse and make me a non-fat latte.

Let's be clear, I was never an athlete of any kind. You won't later discover that I had a career as a professional field hockey player until I tragically broke my ankle in downhill skiing exhibition to bring the Olympics back to Lake Placid. (LP 2026!!!) I have never, ever run a marathon or regularly participated in weekend games of pick-up basketball. Pick-up cake, yes. Basketball, no.

In fact, I was a nerdy, cello-playing, theatre kid regularly picked last in gym class. I dropped out of the swim team after one practice session. I don't like to sweat. And I've never gotten any satisfaction from limping around on aching legs from "intense quad reps."

I'm not being paid to write this. No one gave me a $10,000 retainer to write an ebook and include their brand in the story. Yes, I will mention the brands by name. (MyFitnessPal, Vivofit, etc) But they worked for me so I thought I should share the specifics.

I am also not here to tell you how much you are going to enjoy this process. It's not fun. You won't feel AMAZING after you successfully run two miles. And you won't LOVE eating salad instead of bread. But you will drop weight. You'll be tired. You will dread the workouts. You'll sneer at your own dinners of sauteed chicken and green beans. However, you will gain a sense of control. You'll understand how terrifyingly wrong you've learned to eat. And how your body will continue to betray you as you get older and older. Yay!

Be warned… I am going to use the word, "fat." I'm not writing this book to mess around with euphemisms like "heavy" or "extra pounds." I don't mean "fat" to be a judgmental term. I was carrying a lot of extra fat. Medically speaking, I had too much body fat. So if you don't like the word fat, you will be offended.

The Timeframe

I want to directly talk about how much time this took, and how I lost 50 pounds between May and November. To begin, I didn't plan on losing 50 pounds in six months. In the past, I had tried to track my weight in the hopes of losing one pound per week for one year. I wasn't tracking calories or exercising at that time, so I after about three months of drawing a line straight across the paper, I gave up.

In April, after three months of semi-regular exercise, I realized my methods were lacking. I had to double my efforts. So, I realistically started this successful plan in May. And there were some delays along the way, as you will see below.

January 2015:
Andrea and I are texting about weight loss and she says, "We've got to get you moving your body."

February - March 2015:
30 minutes of dancing every other day. Occasionally riding a bike around the city for 45 minutes.

April 2015:
Weigh in at doctor: 267 pounds. That was a weight gain of at least 5 pounds.

May 2015:
40-50 minutes of dancing every day at home

June 2015:
Friend visits for two weeks. Exercise drops off, eating out increases. Luckily no weight gain. But probably no weight loss.

July - September 2015:

Started running 3 miles twice per week. Still dancing every other day. In August, I run my first 5K.

October 2015:
I go on a two week vacation during which I likely lost two pounds due to exercise and moderate eating. Running increases to every other day with a minimum of 5 miles.

November 2015:
Scale at home says 215 pounds. (To be accurate it was in kilograms and it said 97 kg.)

The doctor's weigh-in in April was mid-day, with clothes but no shoes. The home weigh-in in May was bone dry and bare naked at home in the morning. Regardless, you can't really argue with the results of going from 267 to 215 between May and November.

Growing Bigger and Bigger

Even when I was thin, I was big. I'm 6'2". It took a lot of eating to turn me from six-foot, 12-year old into a six-foot, two-inch, 19-year old. And during those seven years of constant growth, I ate whatever I wanted, whenever I wanted. I fondly remember borrowing my father's car (several times per week) to go get a Friendly's Reese's Peanut Butter Cup Sundae. The big one.

In college, Friday night was movie night at home. I would make a giant pot of pasta with meat sauce and watch an Alfred Hitchcock movie. After eating a portion of pasta and meat sauce as big as my head, I would haul out the Breyer's Mint Chip and eat until I couldn't feel my tongue. And at that time in my life, I was thin and never had to worry about gaining weight.

Growing boys can eat. A lot. And it ruins us.

So I effectively spent the my first 25 years eating my way through life. Pasta, ice cream, cake, hamburgers, sausages... Anything I wanted. Anything.

And between 25 and 30 I gained a little weight. I filled out. But I was happily fixing up a house in San Diego and working two jobs, so I didn't have the time to think about my waist. I had to buy size 34 jeans instead of 32. So what? I was under 30 years old. After buying a new pair of 34-waist Levi's, I probably went to the food court at the mall and got an ice cream.

Then 30 Happened

30 was the beginning of the end. And the start of a ten year journey that I am hoping ends with this plan. I expect that, soon enough, I'll find myself squarely in the middle of another Oz-like terror show called "Mid-Forties." But I'll walk that yellow brick road when I come to it.

Let's begin with Joey in the Fat Suit. It's the perfect example of one of my clues, or signs, that I needed to make a significant change. In the sitcom, Friends, there is a very brief scene at the end of one episode in which they show an alternative universe, and Joey is fat. Yes, I know everyone remembers Monica in the Fat Suit, but I am a man and so Joey made a bigger impression on me.

And so. Ha ha. Joey in the Fat Suit. Almost as funny as Monica in the Fat Suit. Isn't it funny to see skinny, beautiful people look fat?

("Make that fat man sing for a nickel Mommy! I wanna see the fattie sing. Fat people are funny because they look funny.")

Around the same time that I noticed Joey in the Fat Suit (on re-runs), I also reconnected with two friends via Facebook -- Mike and Peter. (Not their real names.) When I saw Mike's recent photo, I instinctively thought, "Holy crap. Is that Mike or the man who ate Mike?" And then I scolded myself. And told myself not to be so judgemental. "And hey, Dylan, don't spend too much time thinking mean thoughts while eating an ice cream cone or the karma monster will come get you." So when I saw Peter's photo, I took a deep breath and thought, "Holy shit! Is that the man who ate Peter?"

So yeah. I poked at the mean bear that is the karma monster.

Simultaneously I also gave a mental nod the the Hollywood make up folks who did a really good job with Joey in the Fat Suit. Peter looked like Peter in the Fat Suit. And the same for Mike. And I thought, "I really don't want to look like Dylan in the Fat Suit."

Another red flag popped up while I was reading a book about near-death experiences. And in several of the reports, people found themselves looking down on their own bodies uncertain as to who they were seeing. They didn't recognize their own bodies! And I thought to myself, "I don't want my first experience in the Forevermore to be the realization that I look like Dylan in the Fat Suit."

Upon my own death, I would much rather accept the everlasting light of love, reunite with relatives who have passed on, and find out if/when aliens built the pyramids. If don't make some changes, when my life passes before my eyes as I review my experiences on Earth with St. Peter (or Mother Gaia), I'll have to relive all those shameful times when I secretly ate a third piece of wedding cake by the DJ table.

Around the same time, I was in complete astonishment of some women I'd known for the majority of my life -- two from high school and one from college. None of them had been athletes. The two women from high school would only walk around the track during gym class. They wouldn't run or play tennis or go swimming. They put on sweats and walked around the track for 30 minutes. Nothing more. And I distinctly recall watching the woman from college jog up a hill and promptly wretch.

Now all three women were running marathons at 40 years old. Not just 5K or 10K races. Not just a walk for a cure. They ran 26.2 miles. I would actually die if I had to do that.

And being the smart-ass I am, I said, "What are they running from?" Aren't I clever? Don't my questions pierce the veil of superficial behaviors?

Now, I realize what they are running from. They are running away from be fat. I don't even believe they (or I) are putting health and longevity first. We don't want to be fat. We don't want to be judged. We want to walk into a store and find clothes that fit.

Aren't I Special?

Yes. You are very special. You're a Super Secret Special Snowflake and it's not fair that you're fat. You've got a slow metabolism. You have a genetic, glandular problem. You're on medication. You hurt your ankle at Six Flags and you can't jog like you used to. "Bullshit, Ron." (Extra points if you know that movie quote.)

You know what? I'm on medication. I had surgery in 2011 that put me in bed for three months.

Blah.
Blah.
Blah.

Let's start with a lovely quote from Pope Francis. God is not "a magician with a magic wand." We exist in a world ruled by science. I don't really care if you think life ends at death or if you believe the spirit lives on as perpetual energy of love. Right now, you and I live in a very physical world with rules of science. Biology, chemistry, physics… Our bodies are creatures of nature.

When I was about 35 (five years ago), I said to myself, "Self, if you accept your body as it is, and you see yourself for the true size that you are, then through acceptance, you will lose weight." I feel dumb just typing that.

If you need a moment to accept who you are. Then put the book down, give yourself a hug, and try to pick up this book within the next five minutes. Don't wait around for five years hoping you'll get a telegraph from your body saying, "I love you too. I accept you too. I release the extra weight now."

That telegraph never came. But something else did arrive by overnight mail -- my special order jeans. I couldn't find my size at Walmart so I had to special order jeans. (My size wasn't at WALMART!!!) Shit.

So to your mother and grandmother and you dog, Princess Pooch of the Poochy Pooches, you are a Super Special Secret Snowflake. To Mother Earth, G-d, Jesus, and Buddah, you're just fat. They love you, but you're fat. And you need to accept the world you live in is one of science. Basically -- losing weight is a matter of math.

Exercise

I started exercising because I didn't want a bag of saline wrapped around my stomach and a port coming out my left side like a water bubbler. Just prior to my first serious attempts at exercise, two close friends opted for stomach reduction/gastric bypass. So I looked into it. I felt a little desperate. I could see Dylan in the Fat Suit in my future, and I wanted to avoid him.

The idea of a surgical solution to a 50 pound problem seemed extreme, but I took the necessary steps to read into the process. And decided against it. One form of weight reduction surgery results in a tube coming out of your body so you can use a saline solution and adjust the size of a sac wrapped around your stomach. Bleck.

Then my friend Andrea said to me, "We need to get you moving." Now Andrea is the sort of woman you pay attention to. When Andrea says, "Jump" you damn well better jump or have the crutches to prove why you couldn't. So I decided to start exercising.

But how much exercise did I need? I had NO clue. However, I consulted a close friend who had worked with a weight loss doctor for several years. He offered a program that required his patients to exercise for seven hours per week. Basically one hour per day doing cardio. I may have actually snorted when she told me that I needed to average one hour per day. Scoffed.

But Andrea said it was time to start moving my body. So I did.

In the past, I had tried bike riding and swimming casually, but neither seemed convenient enough for me to do on a semi-regular basis. Plus, in France, to swim in a municipal pool, you have to wear a skin-tight suit and bathing cap. I took issue with feeling like a white whale in a speedo, so swimming was out. Biking seemed too lackadaisical -- as if I would need a baguette and bouquet of flowers in the basket or I would get kicked off the road.

However, back in the day (a la 1993), my mother kept her pounds off with Richard Simmons and Dancin' to the Oldies. And although my living room was the size of most American closets, I decided it was time to create my own Dancin' routine.

Laundry has always been one of the primary reasons I detest working out. You're left with all those icky, sweaty clothes to wash and dry. So instead of working out in gym clothes, I danced naked.

WARNING: Brief nudity ahead.

Honestly, the naked dancing was a great start. And three close friends asked if there was too much flopping around. Many men shrink, so there really isn't much to flop around in an air conditioned living room. (Even with weak-ass French air conditioning.)

And while you might not need clothes, you do need music. Don't try to exercise without music. It doesn't work. My internet connection in France would frequently grind to halt every day -- often while I was dancing. And when the internet froze, I lost my streaming YouTube music videos. Dancing naked in silence feels a lot more like Silence of the Lambs than Dancin' to the Oldies.

You can easily create a YouTube playlist of your favorite songs. Mostly I picked hits from the 80s and girl-power songs. Probably because they really encourage positive change. Regardless, my "you-go-girl" music did the trick.

- "Shake It Off"
- "You Can't Stop the Beat"
- "Queen of the Night"

Up tempo stuff to keep me moving.

I would set the kitchen timer for 32 minutes and dance like a maniac every other day. And after six weeks, I had gained weight. I. Had. Fucking. Gained. Weight. WTF?

Life is not a Pie Eating Contest

You can exercise on a regular basis. You can track what you eat. But until you do both together, you won't lose weight. Here's why.

Weight loss is science. If you don't remember why, re-read the part above about the Pope and God's magic wand. Weight loss is calories in vs. calories out. And you need to know both numbers to understand how and why you will lose weight.

Technically, you don't need to exercise to lose weight. You could reduce your caloric intake by roughly 500 or 600 calories below your daily "minimum" and yes, you would lose weight. But right now, you're eating more than your minimum. If you were only eating the minimum, you wouldn't be fat. You continue to eat too much. (FYI... the minimum is called your Basal Metabolic Rate and you can read more about it in the back of the book.)

So not only do you have to reduce your caloric intake below minimum, you have to reduce it down to minimum first. And if you are anything like me, you have no idea how much is too much.

And who's to blame?
1. Mom - because she fed you huge portions of butter-rich food.
2. Grandma - because she made delicious chocolate chip cookies.
3. Dairy Queen - because their ice cream is impossibly smooth. (How do they do that?)

No. Mom and Grandma and Dairy Queen are not at fault. It's your body's fault. Your body spent 21 years telling you to "EAT! EAT! EAT!" like you were in the lead at a county pie eating contest. Your body took in hamburgers and sausages and Dairy Queen cones like

Armageddon was three days away. And then, your body got you successfully to age 36 or 38 and said, "job done." We can die now.

Keep in mind, our bodies are designed (by whatever deity you pray to) to keep us alive long enough to see our genes move on. That doesn't just mean by one generation, but two. Our bodies know that it's more important to help raise a grandchild than to raise a child. (Because LORD KNOWS that new mommas need some help with the babies!)

Once we have been old enough to pass our genes through two caveman generations (first at 15 with the birth of our own children, and then at 30 with the birth of our grandchildren), then our body is ready for the great Dairy Queen in the sky.

Awww but look. You're 40. Genetically, you're useless. But you're still eating like a horny 17-year old hoping to have another five or six babies.

So let's look at OPTION 1 -- reduce, reduce, reduce. Do you remember the ads that said, "A shake for breakfast. A shake for lunch. And a sensible dinner." Here's how that translates. "250 calories. 250 calories. 500 calories." And with those rates, you'd probably drop two pounds per week.

Have you ever tried to live on 1,000 calories. By the end of the day, you're standing in your kitchen eating hot dog rolls with cream cheese and wondering why no one ever made French-dressing flavored potato chips.

1,000 calories per day is a nightmare. Go ahead. Try it. I'll wait here.

How'd that go? About as well as hanging wallpaper with your significant other. (True story -- "How the fuck do you hold down a job when you can't hold up a piece of paper?")

A shake for breakfast, a shake for lunch, and a sensible murder at dinner. Your body simply can't turn off the "FIND FOOD" switch when you only eat 1,000 calories per day.

Frankly, at 1,000 calories per day, you're probably not eating enough protein anyway. (See the section about the food groups.) So OPTION 1 is fairly useless.

OPTION TWO is exercise. I know you hate it. It's OK. I do too. But I hate being fat just slightly more than I hate exercise.

I started to see the logic behind the exercise program that requires seven hours of exercise per week. And (as it turns out) a calorie reduction far below the minimum.

So for the science to work, I had to burn, on average, 600 calories per, day. PLUS I had to reduce my caloric intake by 200 calories per day. After 25 weeks, I lost 50 pounds. That's two pounds per week.

I now have three options for exercise. 1) Dancing naked 2) Bike riding, 3) Running. As mentioned before, I've started running. Frankly, I wasn't ready when I started, and I hurt my knees. After one particularly bad run, a physician friend said I would immediately need the legs removed at the hips. I opted to wait. Eventually the Advil kicked in and my legs were saved. But for a brief moment, I saw the beauty of having a legitimate excuse to sit on my ass all day for the rest of my life.

Losing weight is about combining well-informed eating choices with sufficient amounts of safe exercise so you can eat a normal amount of food on a regular basis.

When you exercise without tracking your calories you are simply giving yourself a fantastic excuse for a peanut butter sundae. And if you don't exercise to lose weight, you simply don't eat enough to stay sane.

Where Does the Fat Go?

Like most people, I had no idea where the fat goes when you lose it. (I had to Google it.) Frankly, it's astonishing.

You exhale it.

At its core, this book is about science and the math of losing weight. So the issue eventually becomes how does the body burn fat? And honestly, I am not a science guy. But here goes…

In the same way your car needs fuel to go further, you body needs fuel to exercise more. And it will use your body fat to give you the energy to exercise. The fat becomes fuel when it get broken up into smaller parts. The oxygen you inhale combines with some of those components and becomes the stuff you exhale.

The scary science looks like this:
When you need energy, fat breaks into glucose (and other stuff)
Glucose + Oxygen = CO_2 + H_2O + Energy (ATP)
(For the record, I have no idea what ATP means. I found this using the Google search, "converting fat to co2".)

As you can see, H_2O (aka, water) is part of how you lose weight. But the science stuff shows that it's only 15% of the weight. So you are exhaling 85% your fat. Weird? Yes. But true.

Your breath has weight because it's made up of molecules. So the more you exhale, the more weight you lose. And you have to do a lot of exhaling to lose 50 pounds. But that's why you need to exercise a lot.

Can you sit around and exhale more? No. That's called hyperventilating and you will pass out. So you really, really just have to get your body moving more so you exhale more.

Exercise is a Habit

Simplicity was key for me within the first three months. I get little to no actual satisfaction out of physical activity. So if there was any kind of deterrent (like laundry or leaving the house), I might have stopped.

Going to the gym took up time and energy. And money. Riding my bike involved putting on my helmet. (Which takes effort.) I needed to create a habit. Psychologically, you have to repeat an act up to thirty times for it to become a habit.

As I already mentioned, I started my exercise routine by dancing every other day for 30 minutes. After several weeks, I found I had gained weight -- mostly because I wasn't tracking my calories. Exercise had become an excuse to eat more.

I kicked myself. I kept thinking, "Had I done this properly, I would already have lost ten pounds. I might as well give up now."

But, I have a friend who has this astonishing ability to ignore any negative thoughts. She's blind to them. Frankly, it's amusing sometimes.

> "Alison, I see you broke your arm. How terrible!"

> "Now, I get to learn to use my left hand for painting and writing and driving my manual transmission car!"

Ugh. So, with Alison in mind, I decided it was best not to view my weeks of useless exercise as useless. Instead, I decided to see it as a form of conditioning -- getting my body ready for more exercise.

Now, I can't be sure, but it's possible that was a valid approach. Keep in mind, I've never been an athlete. I've had a moderately distant relationship with my body for my entire life. My body tolerates me and I tolerate it. So thrusting myself into a daily hour of exercise could have been problematic.

In order to lose weight, you have to think about exercising as often as you think about eating. And you have to exercise six out of seven days. You eat everyday, so you should be exercising nearly that often. I like to think about exercise in the same way I think about eating yogurt. I eat yogurt everyday. Maybe one in every ten days will go by when I don't have yogurt. (Keep in mind I am a vegetarian, so yogurt is one of my primary sources of protein.) What do you eat everyday? Toast? Eggs? Radishes? You should be exercising as often as you eat that food.

Limiting your calories and exercising everyday is a physical and mental shift. You have to change the way you eat and how frequently you move your body.

If you've never been physically active, and you're over 20 years old, be prepared for some pushback by your body parts. For example, after dancing for several weeks, I developed tennis elbow. (No. I wasn't playing tennis.) My right elbow just started aching regularly. Still does.

I had started with 30 minutes of dancing every other day. But when I started to track my calories, I started dancing everyday for 40 minutes. Then 50 minutes.

Finally, I decided to go for a run. And let me tell you, that felt like being possessed. Who was I? A runner?

Running, however, when done responsibly, burns an extraordinary number of calories in a short period of time. But at a cost.

To start, I put on my heavy, expensive hiking sneakers and ran three miles. Frankly, I was shocked that I ran that far. Effectively, I had done the Couch to 5K program without knowing it. There is no way that I could have run 5 kilometers (3.1 miles) had I not spent three months dancing daily in my living room. My legs had built up some muscle and were ready for a new challenge.

So I bought a pair of affordable running shoes and pressed forward.

Holy cow was THAT a mistake. After three or four runs in my $15 shoes my knees felt ruined. Luckily I had an aunt that wanted to help me with my fitness goals and she bought me some shoes and fitness monitor to guide me along the way.

All the Extras

Frankly, you don't need to buy anything. To lose weight, you simply need to dance in your living room. Sure, you need some music and a towel. But, as I said, you don't even need clothes.

After using my fitness tracking devices, I compared my actual calorie usage to the estimated calorie count from MyFitnessPal. Nearly the same. According to MyFitnessPal, 50 minutes of naked dancing burns 778 calories. My fancy fitness tracker and heart rate monitor says I lose (on average) 790 calories dancing for 50 minutes.

My aunt Laura bought me a Garmin Vivofit system and expensive Nike running shoes. The expensive running shoes are absolutely critical if you want to push your fitness routine to include jogging. Otherwise you'll lose the use of your knees.

I appreciate the Vivofit system, but I have to emphasize that this kind of body-adorning fitness paraphernalia is not necessary. (Just track your calories. Dance (naked!) for 50 minutes everyday.) However, because the focus of my fitness efforts was on the science behind my weight loss, I was happy to have some specific data via the Vivofit.

Primarily, the Vivofit gives me an idea of my heart rate while I exercise. I use it while I am running and dancing. I can start to see the ways in which heart rate effects calorie burn, and I have started making some small adjustments during my routines to speed up or slow down my heart rate. Actually, when I am running, I don't really need to heart rate monitor to tell me when to slow down; the urge to bend over and vomit is usually the sign that I am pushing myself too far. However, thanks to Vivofit, I know that when my heart rate reaches 178 beats per minute, my body wants to wretch.

Using the Scale

Don't use the scale. It's not your friend. You've heard this advice before, but here's why. When you are losing weight at a rate of two pounds per week, you will be losing about one-quarter of a pound per day. That's not going to show up on any scale. And there are too many other body variables to influence your overall weight.

Let's break down the numbers. One-quarter of a pound is a half-cup of water (8 ounces). You won't even pee if you have 8 ounces of water in your bladder. A cup of coffee or a neglected toenail will throw off your daily losses on the scale.

WARNING: POTTY TALK AHEAD.

We all go through the pre-weighing ritual. Of course, you weigh yourself in the morning. After a good poop. And a long pee. Maybe you will pass some gas to reduce any internal pressure that could create extra downward pressure on the scale. Obviously, you only get on the scale when you are buck naked. Hell, I've even brushed my hair before getting on the scale.

The best and worse place to get weighed is at the doctor's office. I always manage to be wearing combat boots on the day I visit the doctor.

> The nurse: No, don't take off your boots for the scale. It's fine.
> Me: Ummm.. it's not fine. The boots are coming off.

But boots or no boots, the doctor's office is actually a good place to get weighed if you are serious about losing 50 pounds in 6 months. Why? Because something like an extra cup of coffee or heavy

Christmas sweater isn't going to obscure losing trackable amounts between your visits to the doctor.

So, go take the batteries out of the bathroom scale right now. It's OK. I'll wait.

Done? LIAR. Go do it.

Seriously, don't weigh yourself at home. You won't really see a difference in your weight. And if you weigh yourself everyday, you'll get discouraged, call me a liar, and give my book a bad review on Amazon.

Don't weigh yourself. Let the doctor do it.

Food Tracking

If daily exercise is the "HOW" of weight loss, then tracking your caloric intake is the "WHY". Unless you keep track of what you eat, you won't lose weight.

[Read the following in an annoying, high-pitched voice.]
"Diet and exercise. Diet and exercise.
[End annoying voice.]

I previously established that trying to reduce your weight by reducing calories simply leads to murdering your loved ones. As I also mentioned, if you only exercise, and you don't track your food intake, you'll justify putting Laura Scudder's All Natural Peanut Butter on Breyer's Chocolate Ice Cream.

Losing weight is a science. You are an animal that operates in a physical world. If you know the numbers, then you can lose the weight. You start making informed decisions because you see where the calories are going. When you properly track your food, you start to realize the bad decisions that have prevented you from losing weight your whole life.

Nuts: Peanuts, walnuts, cashews… say good-bye. They will soak up an entire day's worth of calories instantly. One minute you are looking at a bowl of peanuts… the next minute, they are gone. "But nuts are healthy!" Uh huh. Nuts are healthy for skinny people. Once day, your nut will come. But for now, it's over.

Butter. Let it go. I personally love butter. But it's not worth the calories. If you enjoy your toast with butter in the morning, your calorie allotment will be gone by dinner time. And you'll be back to murdering family members. I can manage to enjoy toast with jam.

Pasta and bread. I held onto these in limited quantities. I couldn't say good-bye. However, I know that I have to put in an extra 20 minutes of exercise when I want pasta for dinner.

Juice. Mostly, no. Juice is a lovely way to start the day, but you can't have more than a half cup. Then it's over. Try freezing the juice in popsicle molds. I find this helps extend the satisfaction lifespan of my half cup serving.

Mayonnaise. HA! You're funny.

I found MyFitnessPal to be the best way to track calories. And I signed up for the premium membership to make the irritating ads go away. (By the way, my MBA compels me to mention I think it's a terrible idea for a company to force customers to spend money so they don't hate the company's website. I'd rather get more useful tools with my premium membership to MyFitnessPal. Thanks.)

Do I think MyFitnessPal perfectly tracks calories? Not really. But I do think that if I enter in all the food I eat, I will be within 50 calories (give or take) of my actual intake. After six months, I can safely say that I have also decreased my food intake because I've determined what foods have the lowest calorie count with the highest satisfaction. For me, nonfat greek yogurt with stevia packets makes for a perfect breakfast and end-of-day snack.

I also like to see what nutrients need the most adjustment. As a vegetarian, I wasn't surprised to see that I didn't get quite enough protein. However, I will say that I don't think enough people get high-quality, low fat protein in their diet.

Fiber is also missing from most of our diets. For long-term health benefits, almost nothing matches a high fiber diet. Unfortunately, fiber comes with carbohydrates, so you need something with dense fiber. There is nothing like Kellogg's All Bran to get you the most fiber BANG for your caloric buck. For those of you who remember the early 1990s Saturday Night Live, you'll recall the Colon Blow ads. That's All Bran. If you choose to add All Bran into your diet, experiment a little. Because when the fiber hits, you have very little time before touchdown.

Skinny People and Calories

Do skinny people have it easier? Yes. And not only do they have higher pay at better jobs, they don't have to watch what they eat as much as you do. Skinny people (SPs) often don't have to exercise to keep their trim waists.

Is it fair? Ummm…. no. But the SPs haven't spent the last ten years eating their way through Thanksgiving and Christmas with excuses like, "But Christmas a birthday party!" The SPs have eaten responsibly for the majority of their lives. And some even exercise. So the ESPs (exercising skinny people) can go for a jog and then eat a giant, 700 calorie sundae. Bitches.

Face Facts: You are in caloric debt. If you want to drop 50 pounds you have burn an additional 175,000 calories in the next six months to even the score.

Yes. 175,000 calories. Every pound of fat is roughly 3,500 calories. In order to cover that kind of ground, you will need to burn 800 extra calories every day over your base calorie rate.

So, either eat 800 fewer calories, or increase the number of calories you burn by exercising. Or a combination of both.

My personal calculation works like this:
Base caloric rate: 2400 per day to maintain body size
Exercise: 700 calories per day
Total allowable calories per day with exercise to MAINTAIN weight: 3100 (woo hoo)

-450 calories per day to lose 1 pound per week
-900 calories per day to lose 2 pounds per week
-1350 calories per day to lose 3 pounds per week

So let's opt for two pounds per week: 3100-900=2200

So if I exercise for 50 minutes everyday, then I can eat 2200 calories per day and lose 2 pounds per week. This is scientific fact. I am proof that this formula works.

2 pounds per week for 26 weeks = 50 pounds in 6 months.

You can set MyFitnessPal to do most of these calculations for you. I suggest setting your MyFitnessPal target to losing 2 pounds per week. Honestly I set mine for 1 pound per week, and then tried to change it half-way through this process. Once you set that goal, don't alter it. You can stray from the goal if you want -- going over or under the calories count -- but once you've lived with the set goal for more than a few weeks, leave it alone. Your brain has to learn. At the moment, you don't understand what a normal day of eating looks like. If you're like me, you never thought much about the cumulative effect of your total daily calories. And it got you fat.

The MyFitnessPal calorie goal is THE way to re-train your brain. You need to give yourself several months of calorie tracking to understand what your body realistically needs everyday. You can't trust your mind, because clearly you've been overeating. And you really can't trust your body -- you've been feeding the body monster for years. It's time to tame the body monster with some hard core facts.

Types of Calories

When it comes right down to the bottom line -- the calories per day bottom line -- a calorie is a calorie is a calories.

"But avocado fat is GOOD fat. Like pecans."

Ummm... sure. And you can have as much of that avocado fat as you want. And when your caloric intake goes over the daily target, you start gaining weight.

"Olive oil fights other fats."
"Juice has vitamin C."
"Studies say you need lots of protein to feel full."

Quack.
Quack.
Quack.

If you eat too many calories, you gain weight.

Calories come in three forms: carbs, protein, and fat. And in this trio, fat and carbs are like siblings. And protein is the third cousin twice removed.

You body wants to use carbs immediately. Like coal going into the steam engine of the train to make the machine go. If your body doesn't use those new carbs immediately, it puts them away in storage -- as fat.

Your body constantly needs fresh protein. It's very difficult for your body to live without new proteins everyday. So when you eat while on a diet, you need to make sure you are getting enough protein. MyFitnessPal has the fantastic feature of showing you exactly how much protein (and fat and carbs and fiber) you are consuming everyday. Watch this number closely. Get as close to the target protein number as possible without going over on the total caloric intake.

Finally, fat. And fat is tricky. You eat fat and oils. You've stored too much fat. But how does fat intake and fat storage relate to carb intake and protein intake. Frankly it's complicated. This is where a lot of the no carb dieting options originate. Atkins, paleo, caveman… these are forms of dieting that manipulate the body into thinking that it's starving. These can be effective. As I type this, a good friend is under a doctor's supervision for a form of the Atkin's diet. There is no problem with these diets, but they don't teach you anything. They simply trick your body.

What I'm saying in this book is that you and I are naive. We've been slowly brainwashed by our mind and body into thinking that we can eat whatever we want like we're 15 years old. I am trying to learn how to eat properly. I don't know what "a lot" of food looks like. I don't know why "exercise matters!".

I've seen my mother and my cousin lose a significant amount of body fat with Atkin's. But that diet is difficult to sustain over a lifetime. Holiday cookies, restaurants, and vacations happen. So unless you want to spend the rest of your life eating only pizza toppings, then you need to learn why you can't have more than two slices of pizza. Or if you do indulge in five slices, why you have to dance naked for 50 minutes to burn it off.

Let's also talk about changing your metabolism.

The package on my box of green tea says it will increase my metabolism. So maybe if you drink enough of the green tea, you won't have to exercise. The green tea will burn off the fat, right?

No.

Legally, the company that makes that weight loss tea needs to show that your body's metabolism will scientifically change with consumption. And technically, they can prove that the claim is scientifically true. However, it's about as true as saying you changed the volume of the ocean when you dump a bucket of water into it. Did it change? Ummmm sure. Does it really make a difference? Not at all.

But if you want to drink your weight loss tea, please do. Then go for a jog.

Interestingly, I am not even sure if exercise will dramatically change your metabolism. In fact, as you lose weight, your allotted number of calories decreases per day. When I started on this diet, I was able to eat 2200 calories per day. After losing 25 pounds, My Fitness Pal downgraded by calories to only 2050. (Fuckers!)

Food and Recipes

Marie Osmond is one of those modern diet icons that comes to mind when I decided to seriously attempt a weight loss program. And in one of her commercials she talks about eating desserts like cake and pudding. Now, Marie Osmond has always been a little scary to me -- along the lines of "No more wire hangers!" And while I would never have had the courage to say it to her face, I doubted that you could eat cake and lose weight. But she's right; you can.

The curse and the beauty of knowing calories in/calories out is that you can make some informed decisions. At the end the book, I've included a sample of one day of food for me. I deliberately chose a sample day in which I ate some cookies.

At the three month mark, I noticed a remarkable downward shift in my calorie intake. Up to that point, I was averaging close to 1900 calories per day, but as I learned which foods had the most impact on my body, I was able to cut down my intake to 1400.

At the same time, I started running. So on several occasions, I burned 1100 calories, but only ate 1400 calories. That's a net of only 300 calories consumed for the day. And with my body naturally burning roughly 2400 calories just to keep the train in motion, I probably had a -2100 calorie day.

Woo hoo!
Yay.
What's wrong?

The morning after one of those -2100 calorie days, I crawled out of bed at 6am and gobbled up a bowl of dry oatmeal soaked in milk. Then I felt nauseated. And some darkness started to creep in around the periphery of my vision. To say that I almost passed out is a touch dramatic; but manipulating your diet comes with a price.

Meal Planning

After spending a few weeks tracking my food intake, I started to pre-plan my eating for the day. This effort did not come out of a sense of responsibility, but naive hope. I'd start with a standard breakfast like oatmeal or yogurt and then I would start thinking that I could skip my exercise regime for the day.

So every day, as if I hadn't done the same EXACT thing for the last several months, I would sit down and pre-enter my food into MyFitnessPal. And everyday, I would look with horror at how many calories I planning on consuming. Only then would I come to the conclusion that if I wanted to have more to eat than the bare minimum, I would have to dance or run.

As I mentioned before, eventually I was able to pare down my calorie intake to roughly 1400 instead of 2100. And as I started running more regularly, I started playing a numbers game with my calories in and calories out.

Sometimes it felt more like running numbers at the track with a bookie instead of running a 5K for personal fitness. "If I dance for 50 minutes today and go for a bike ride to the beach, then I can have croissant in the morning. But then I have to go for a run, so that I can eat all that pasta for dinner tomorrow."

But planning your food intake is also a good way to put your food obsession to use. When I wasn't watching anything but my waist grow bigger, I frequently spent many happy hours daydreaming about upcoming dinners at Miguel's in San Diego or trips to Yogurtland with my mother (where she always ordered too much and I had to finish her dish and mine).

Now, I could look forward to food, but in less exciting ways. Yay, a smoothie at 3pm. Quiche at 7pm. And more Greek yogurt at 10pm!

Part of weight loss science is teaching your mind what to expect throughout the day. It might not be as good as thinking about freshly made flour tortilla chips with jalapeno cream salsa, but it's better than feeling confused why the weight won't come off. (As if the cream salsa wasn't a clue.)

One of my favorite features of MyFitnessPal is the Recipes tool. As I mentioned, I cook most of my own food. Plus, I don't eat much prepared food. Without the Recipe tool, this might make counting my calories difficult. The tool allows you to enter the ingredients of your recipe and indicate the number of serving. Then, you can save and log the custom food.

Sleep

At the start of this diet endeavor, I was an overweight, non-athletic 40 year old man. Even during the firsts few months when I was only exercising every-other day for 30 minutes, the exercise was taking a toll on my body. Once I upped the rate to 50 minutes every day, my body nearly went into shock.

"Exercise will enervate you!"
"You'll have MORE energy."
"You'll jump out of bed every morning!"

No, no, and no. I was tired. And not just during the ten hours of sleep I needed. I was tired during the day sometimes. However, physical exhaustion (a little extreme, I admit) feels very different from sleep deprivation. I never had the urge to nap. I wasn't falling asleep while watching reruns of Friends.

Mostly, my body seemed confused. As I've said, I've never been much of an athlete. I never had an urge to kick a ball on a field or run around a court of any kind. Honestly, I think athletes get some sort of real satisfaction out of this feeling of physical exertion. I don't get it. But, that doesn't matter.

When you're in caloric debt, you've got to set aside enough time to exercise and sleep.

Even the most casual of athletes probably have some sort of working knowledge of recovery time. Parents, coaches, friends… the physically active have several sources of information about how to recover from fitness activities. I never had a reason or an interest in the topic.

It would be like trying to get my athletic father to have an active conversation about the parallels between Goldie Hawn, Mira Sorvino, and Jennifer Lawrence winning Oscars at such a young age. You'd get dead silence. Crickets. Tumbleweed rolling by.

If you've never been physically active, you probably don't have even the most basic knowledge of how to responsibly exercise. However, this is not an excuse to avoid the ugly reality of sweat. Your body was made to move. So move it.

You will feel aches and pains. Obviously, if there are stabbing pains or extreme aches, use common sense and stop. Please don't sue me because you broke your foot while dancing in your living room and didn't go to a doctor. When you start using your body, keep using your head.

Getting Started (and Losing the Weight)

1) Create a MyFitnessPal account.
2) Use it. Set your weight loss goal and stick to the calorie count.
3) Create a music playlist. (I used YouTube.)
4) Put a towel down on the living room floor and dance for an hour every day.

That's it. Dance and track your calories.

Everyday.

The Fallout

A successful diet might put a strain on some of the closest relationships in your life. And some of that strain will come from you, and some will come from your friends and family. Change is difficult. For everyone.

You will see people react. Changing your size shifts the balance of how people see themselves in relation to you. Husbands, wives, lovers, sisters, mothers, etc… they will all react, as will you. Some will take your change as a motivation for themselves; as I did when Andrea dropped her weight. Some will talk about it. Others won't. Be proud of your efforts and carry on regardless of how you and those close to you react.

You:
Frankly, you might become one of those tiresome people that talks about calories and exercise. You might suddenly find yourself at a party bonding with some skinny, white woman over running shoes. Or being the first to say no to dessert.

Once you start losing weight, you will be working really, really hard at accomplishing something most people struggle to do. You have new skills and abilities that give you power over your weight. It's like a superpower. So use your powers for good.

The Lovers:
After the three month mark, my weight loss was noticeable. Unfortunately, most of my friends could only see me on Skype and the loss was less apparent. However, thanks to some shameless self-promotion on Facebook, I got some words of encouragement.

To be honest, I always look at positive comments with a jaded view. As if the person might be saying, "Good job!" when he or she really means, "Oh shut up and go back to eating cake." And that's just a form of my own negativity worming its way into my head through any means possible.

Overall, I found that almost everyone was really supportive of my weight loss. And many were willing to ask about my means and methods. Fewer people wanted to know about my running habit, which I took to being a sign that the interest in my weight loss was genuine and true, while no one wants to hear they should run. Most people think about losing weight while, but fewer people are willing to put feet on the ground in a running shoe. And I don't blame them.

One friend in particular was very supportive of both the weight loss and the exercise habits. She has always been thin and fit. In high school she was a sprint runner and is currently the manager of a fitness studio in San Diego. She was that one person who actually said, "Don't you feel SO MUCH better after you exercise? Physically and mentally!" It was then that I really understood that there is a physical difference between me and those who love sports and exercise. Basically, my answer to her was, "No."

I admit that some of my depressive feeling remained at bay once I started exercising. And after being on vacation for one week without any extended physical activity, I found some of my depression creeping back in. But as I've said, I don't have a love of physical fitness. My compulsion is exercise is only slightly greater than my distaste for being overweight.

The Haters:
You might encounter one or two people who want to dwell on some negative aspect of your weight loss. I decided this negativity was an indication of their state of mind. I sympathize with the haters. It's easy to compare yourself to others and ask what you could be doing

differently. And I think it's natural for some form of competition or comparison to arise.

But when you encounter a hater, shift the focus to the now. I have a natural fear that I will regain the weight I've lost. So focusing on my past size (with one of those haters) just gives weight (no pun intended) to the kinds of negative thoughts that can pull you back down.

For example, one person asked me, "So were you really over 260 pounds last year?" It might sound (somewhat) harmless, but it's a fairly straightforward insult. I think it's fair to translate that into, "I can't believe how fat you were!"

As another example, I was sitting in a restaurant with very good friend when he pointed to a man sitting alone at the bar. The guy at the bar looked like an heavy, gay, Hercule Poireau. If he didn't have a twirly moustache and yippy dog, then he should have. "You were headed towards looking like that." Ummmmm… no I wasn't. Even if I was the same weight as that man, I would never take on such an affected appearance.

For some people, weight is a major determinant in how they see others. That's their view of the world.

I say this: people of all sizes are gorgeous. Everyone can be sexy and exciting. Maybe not sexy and exciting to everyone, but to someone. So regardless of your size, be happy with yourself. My self-image hasn't shift as much as my weight. I've lost 20% of my body fat, but I don't see myself as 20% better. I'm still me, and I like myself as much now as I did before.

The Won't Say Much-ers

Lastly, you will encounter the folks who don't mention your weight loss. I struggled with this. I admit it might be hypocritical of me to say it, but if you are one of my best friends, don't ignore this massive change. Say something -- positive or negative.

I also understand that if someone can't think of something nice to say, then the choice to say silent is appropriate.

Andrea and I compared notes on this issue. And she had a more dramatic weight loss than I did. We agreed: saying nothing might be someone way of avoiding an insult to the way I used to look. "Wow! You look great!" might imply that I at one point I didn't look great. So I give a tentative pass to those who might have an internal conflict and chose to say nothing.

Sample Calorie Count

	Calories	Carbs	Fat	Protein	Fiber	Chol
Breakfast						
Cream - Half and half, 0.2 cup	63	2	6	1	0	18
Non Fat Greek Yogurt, 170 g	97	7	0	17	0	7
Total	160	9	0	17	0	7
Lunch						
Soy Milk 230.0 ml	99	2	6	9	0	0
Soy Protein, 0.5 serving	54	0	1	12	0	0
Berries, 0.5 cup	40	0	0	0	0	0
Mangos, raw, 0.25 cup	25	6	0	0	1	0
Total	218	8	6	22	1	0
Dinner						
Salad dressing, 1 serving	166	7	16	0	0	0
Salad, 1 serving(s)	42	9	2	2	3	0
Barilla - Sauce, 0.5 cup	70	14	1	2	3	0
Barilla - Tortellini, 115 g	457	62	15	16	7	0
Total	735	91	34	20	13	0
Snacks						
Cookies w/ Chocolate	191	21	10	3	2	0
Non Fat Greek Yogurt, 158.9 g	91	6	0	16	0	7
Total	282	27	10	19	2	7
Daily Totals	**1,395**	**136**	**56**	**79**	**15**	**32**

Your Daily Calorie Goal is 2050.
You've earned 1,117 extra calories from exercise today.

Your Daily Goal	3,167	396	105	158	38	300
Remaining	1,772	260	49	79	22	267
	Calories	Carbs	Fat	Protein	Fiber	Chol

Basal Metabolic Rate Examples

Male, Age 21, Weight 200:   1,950 calories per day
Female, Age 21, Weight 150:   1,478 calories per day

Male, Age 40, Weight 200:   1,844 calories per day
Female, Age 30, Weight 150:   1,383 calories per day

Male, Age 70, Weight 200:   1,705 calories per day
Female, Age 70, Weight 150:   1,233 calories per day

These calories go towards keeping your body operating. In fact, you can lie in bed all day and you will burn these calories just because your heart is beating and your brain is thinking. So you can always add a few additional calories if you walk around a bit. However, don't add many. Frankly, if you spend a Saturday watching movies and snacking, you will only burn about 100 calories going from the TV to the fridge all day.

direct email:
dylansebooks@gmail.com

website:
www.dylanonline.com

Facebook Page:
https://www.facebook.com/50pounds6months

Facebook Group (The Best Choice!):
https://www.facebook.com/groups/1641314272806119/

Printed in Great Britain
by Amazon